# The Grave Decade

## by

I0426354

## Elisha  Otieno

# DEDICATION

I dedicate this book to my mother Teresia Aluoch Otieno who embraced my family at the time I was struggling for its production.

I dedicate the book to our child hood academic heroes who were disappointed by circumstances beyond control like Jobic Odembo and Joseph Okare.

Finally, I dedicate this book to my third follower Joseph Juma who developed health complications similar to mine at the age of only two and died more than two decades later at the age of twenty six years.

For direct comments to the Author,send to:-
Email: aribatec@gmail.com

# TABLE OF CONTENTS

# PREFACE

The Grave Decade is a self testimonial non fiction story book written to share my personal experience of ten years in infirmity with the world after keen analysis and conclusion that it was indeed necessary for the benefit of other victims of similar calamities. The book covers a wide range of challenges involved including social, religious and development intricacies one faces when in a situation that creates a wedge between you and the surrounding community. My earlier decision to dunk my head under the water to keep it a secret was disapproved by several victims of other health complications including the Kenyan Minister for Medical Services Professor Peter Anyang Nyongo who publicly shared his experience in prostate cancer. The pain is soothed by ridiculous encounters that are relish able to any reader who loves interesting stories. One of the most important lessons from the book is the anti hospital religious doctrines as viewed from my personal experience. My endeavor to write was infused by the Writers Bureau-Manchester-England where I registered as a student in 2010.

As a new breed of fish in the lake of writers, I felt rejuvenated when my first article *Dialogue Saves Kenya* was published by a Canadian magazine~*Pages of Stories-A special war edition* in 2011 and decided to take it a notch higher by writing this book. I am flexing my muscles to write fictions that reflect our day to day life experiences aimed at offering lessons in a way or another. I wish you enjoyable reading.

**Elisha Otieno**
**Siaya-Kenya**
Email: aribatec@gmail.com

# ACKNOWLEDGEMENT

Erick Odiang'a of Siaya Kenya Computers is the father and founder of my writing career. He single handedly sacrificed to pay for one hundred presale copies of this book to pave way for full production of the book as per our contract agreement with the publisher. May God bless pastor Paul Odiel of Skills for Living church-Siaya for introducing me to Mr Odiang'a and assisting to win his trust.

My gratitude goes to Samuel Oloo of Orient Educational Centre-Siaya for his incautious contribution to finance the administration fees required for the work of this book to commence.

*"The wealth of our graves swells high from the harvest of unripe fruits. The gawky angel of death gawks at the medicine man with pain. He whines and writhes in bitterness at the crisis. Health solution is a crisis...! To him, it's a crisis. The grave digger growls in his spirits. Cure is a crisis...!. To him, it's a crisis. It's a scarcity....!, a scarcity of job, a scarcity of bread and butter. His business blossoms, with the caravan of souls leaving the surface of the seventh planet".*

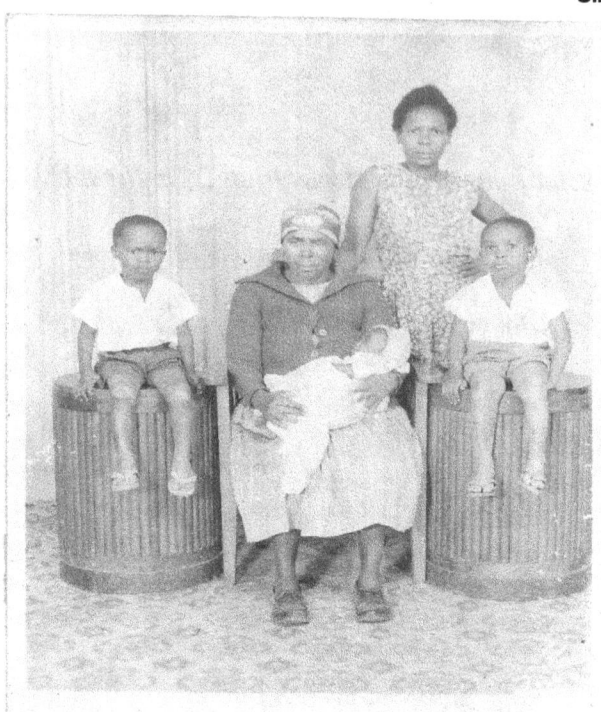

Five months old Elisha Otieno (carried by granny),his
mother(Standing),Siblings-Isaack Onyango (seated right) and
Tobias Otieno-*Tobby*(Seated left)

# CHAPTER ONE

A strange electronic sensation in my nervous system worsened by a rhythm of pounding beats on my almost exploding head like a slam of hammer from an assailant, a trail of saliva dribbling from my mouth down to the mattress like spilled milk, pain from my lower lips damaged by teeth marks, evidently from several vigorous bites and bruises from my fists, feet, shoulder and other external parts of my body unveils some grisly scenario of a battle between me and some powerful forces, but when and how is the question that lingers in my mind.

The night this happened, my siblings and I had retired to bed as was our lifestyle during the 1980s.All the male grandchildren from the different families that composed the home of our grandparents would dine together and sleep in a house reserved for the purpose .The females shared the house with the old mother of our fathers to keep her happy .There was no sign of health complications when I joined the rest on the extended family bed to sleep.

I tried to lift my head but my neck muscles contracted involuntarily rendering my efforts useless. I collapsed back to the bed in exhaustion and my groggy body relaxed hopelessly.

A tune of a worship song mostly used in funerals and sorrowful occasions found its way into my ears blowing my memories more closer to the grave than just the health conditions. The singers, a group of pious relatives arched around my bed conclusively caressed my numb body, wiped the saliva spills and placed me in a good sleeping position. A comment from one of them gnawed a big portion of my heart "may be it's a demon of epilepsy?". The last word floored my hopes, on imaginations of the vicissitudes of the deadly nervous disease as I knew it from other victims.

I fell into a deep slumber and woke up hours later with some strength to at least stagger out of the bed, muscle cramps still at their peak, no munchies for any delicacies, my nerves bent by frustrations. Gasping for breath with pain, I moved to a secluded site under a mango tree to bask in the afternoon sunshine that I had missed for long hours. Everybody gawping at me from a distance. Experienced elderly observers occasionally paying visits for words of encouragement but trimming their words never to tell me what exactly they had discovered about the new development in my life.

\* \* \*

# FIRST AID

The bright sunshine, a few degrees past center, blinded my eyes. Under normal circumstances, today being a school holiday, I would be part of a team enjoying bull fights at the grazing field and trying to prove our manhood by talking sweet nothings to females of our age who were fetching firewood at the same venue. But unfortunately the spirits of a bad omen had launched a phenomenon that would take years to understand and come to grips with. Granny and Steve, her eldest son held me by the shoulders and whispered words of encouragement to me. Together they lifted me up and let me try to balance but I crumbled back. Steve burst into uncontrollable sobs, but granny reprimanded him for mourning a person who was alive. They carried me to a fenced bathing place and gave me a forced bath. I resisted because letting somebody wash me at the age of fourteen was an affront to my virility.

The two care takers had diverging opinions on the first medication. While Steve applied *"sloans"*, a medical solution used for bone injuries rubbed on my chest, granny applied hot water mixed with herbal solutions to my joints. I felt like somebody had off loaded a tank of water from my chest. I felt my stomach gnawing with at least some appetite for food restored. I emptied the steaming calabash of fermented porridge from granny's ever flowing pot.

\*\*\*

# FACING THE REALITY

With my senses reactivated back to normalcy, I sat on a creaky chair at a corner of my granny's main house to account for every detail of my movements before the fateful night. Rumours had already swirled around the village and curious visitors were flocking in and treating me with the kind of respect I didn't deserve to express their grievances. Judging from their sympathetic looks and elegiac remarks, I realized the situation was worse than I imagined.

According to granny's earlier stories concerning epilepsy and the circumstances surrounding its victims, it is a satanic force that embroils people who had offended it in a way or another as a penalty for their offences. The evil spirits fear the offenders themselves but they can bounce onto a person of close blood relationship to the offender like his child, wife, grand child or anybody within their genealogical structures.

If a relative dies from the problem, the spirits of epilepsy don't die but they resurrect to haunt another person in the same family lineage.

She explained further that experienced people whose families were affected could collaborate with powerful witchdoctors and by means of their charms divert the spirits to unsuspecting families whose relationship with them was frosty. The charms were sprayed at the path where the target mostly used and once he passed, he could become a victim.

Granny's questionnaire was driving me closer to what I feared most. Although she never called the spade by its name, she asked me questions like if I ever saw any liquid sprayed on my way the day before. Her words burnt like acid, I declined to answer but collected some irksome data.

A bitter pill to swallow lay on my tongue; accepting epilepsy as part of my life. The curse of all curses. My memories ran on several cases in the village and at school and summed up what it entails to live with the merciless assailant who plants his grenades inside the victim's blood circulatory system.

Ugly scenarios of fellow pupils attacked in class and play fields that sent our colleagues wailing themselves hoarse. The stigma experienced by the victims as a result of myths linked to epileptics. The effects resulting from physical injuries with others ending up with disabilities, deaths in water, fire, mental complications developed by some who had stayed with the problem for long durations and all dehumanizing stuff of the enemy sent my hopes packing.

Just before concluding my sad meditation, a boy of my age sidled towards my seat and whispered to my ears "our mother has informed us that as from today, we should not allow you to accompany us to the stream when going to bath"
"Why"
"Because you may die in water, "he answered
A trail of tears rolled down my cheeks. It was already concluded and sealed.

While still meditating on whether it was true or false. Words of precautions were spreading around the village. Uncle Steve's approach was more accommodating. He informed me that he had a dream that I was chosen to be a servant of God and according to the Old Testament, servants of God were not allowed to bath in streams or in open places. He added that because of the respect I deserved, I needed not to go near fire places or walk alone to long distances. I responded with a wry smile but having known his aim, I kept mum.

A week later, I was fully healed physically but the trauma of the incident continued to affect my mind like chicken pox on the skin. Worst of all, the precautions undertaken created a wedge between me and my colleagues in all areas reached with the sad news.

# CHAPTER TWO

I joined the rest in celebrating our last year of primary school education in the wake of the new year after long December holidays.Undoubtebtedly, I'd emerge either best or one of the top if I maintained my position as per earlier records and more better that I was to repeat the class after failing to get school fees in my first attempt in 1987. We bare footedly competed through the labyrinths of the long grass dominated heel leading to the school to avoid the wrath of sturdy prefects deployed at the gate to shower late goers with countless strokes.

***

## THE GRACE YEAR

The first quarter of the year went smoothly without drama, although Wandulo, our school Head Teacher handled me with a gesture likely to suggest that he had a clue. He refined his utterances to encourage than to console. I maintained the top position in all exams and the report seemed to have affected the school administration on why the bad omen on their best performer.

Memories of the past year incident disappeared like vapour.The undocumented laws enacted to guard my movements were flawed. I mingled freely with my peers, went herding and bathing in the streams, swimming and enjoying all sorts of childhood activities of our times.

Wandulo was too aggressive to let a day go without a lesson for the candidates. In the midst of our busy schedule, he voluntarily released us one Saturday afternoon to go and view a python that had been killed near a bush across the stream. I developed cold feet on our way back when my scared classmates were fleeing from a herds boy who went into convulsions leaving his cattle to roam freely.

With a lump in my throat, I gravitated towards his direction and started sobbing near him as if attracted by some magnetic forces until his relatives arrived at the scene to rescue. I felt too discouraged to go back to school. Wandulo who had been tipped by my colleagues took me to his office for some counseling and encouragement the following day when I reported back. I maintained my studies despite the setback, a feeling that kept on reminding me that life was meaningless if I had to leave with the disease.

On humanitarian grounds, Wandulo informed his staff members about my state and advised them not to apply tough measures in their punishments any time I went astray. The prefects avoided me while exercising their powers on malingerers during pre-parade manual work time. Whenever I had wrangles with other pupils, they would resort to humble themselves by pleading guilty and running away than fighting somebody whose health condition was treated with sympathy. Worst of all, ceremonial activities like village discos, interschool sports where I'd meet polite rejections whenever I tried to join others in rejoicing especially toying around with girls; our gauge of manhood.

I threw my pride to the wind and embarked on studies. Even though my academic performance remained high, I still felt I was pissing the wind "who'll ever employ me after all in that state?" I surrendered from the jovial community lifestyle to a new description; a forlorn sickly, sombre boy.

\*\*\*

## FIRST ENCOUNTER WITH THE EXORCIST

Mesmerizing other victims whenever they were attacked were too traumatizing for me and our entire family to assume all was well. My problem was shared with anybody who promised to have a solution.

A woman Pentecostal who claimed to have powers to drive out the evil spirits invited me to their overnight evil spirits battling spree scheduled to take place at her home.

The warm glow of the setting sun spilled through the vegetation on the parallel landscape into the house providing a conducive atmosphere for our preparatory meeting. I joined a group of religious leaders clad in their church gowns and caps adorned with the symbol of the cross. On the table at the centre of the room was the crucifix propped against a stand designed for the purpose and surrounded by lit candles believed to have some spiritual influence depending on their colors.

Only subjects of the night's prayer sessions were allowed to share the table with the spiritual fathers and spill their guts before joining the rest. I tried to jog away the jitters as more spirited men and women of God bowed at the door before stepping into the hallowed floor of the room occupied by the clergy and their catch. When the floor was packed, the meeting was flagged off after a short prayer.

The victims, referred to as the *possessed* sat on one side of the table facing the servants of God. Each of us had to spill the beans on how exactly *"your enemy"* according to their language works. A girl seated at the edge of our bench testified about persistent stomach ache. Next to her just before me was a man whose case was mental and his mother chose to speak on his behalf. A preacher glared at me accusingly when my turn came, asking condemning questions like "what did your people do for such a bad spirit to establish a home in you?" The last casualty who spoke after me had a petty issue, he used to feel pain in his eyes whenever he tried to read.

We left the house and joined the multitude of the laity and observers who thronged the home of our host for spiritual deliverance. Majority were dressed in church attires of varying colors depending on the angel you represented according to the denominational belief that every angel identified by their names like Gabriel was attracted to a particular color apart from the newcomers who were in their civilian clothes.

The full bright moonlight hovering from the cloudless blue sky shone over a sea of humanity seated on the bare grass in the open compound listening to the church leaders immediately before flagging off the spiritual battle aimed at the cases presented before the holy table. Gigantic kettles of scalding hot tea were served to the congregation to keep the cold overnight wind at bay.

The spiritual strongman's speech was severally interrupted by growls and shouts of tongues from staunch believers filled with the Holy Ghost responding to calls from the spirit world. I found myself in unfamiliar grounds and felt like crawling on my knees to sneak and go back home with my grunge. The Holy Father's speech itself was condemning, too condemning to give room for explanation, otherwise, I could explain that I was not responsible for the sins of my forefathers. I obeyed his order that the casualties of the day to go on their knees arched around the clergy's table and lift their spirits close to the Heavenly Father, my knees did but my spirits declined, lacking the ladder to use, instead I kept wondering in fear how the night would be with powerful angelic messengers of God performing spiritual war activities on me.

A long quite low tone worship song greased the occasion, followed by vigorous drumbeats and loud songs performed by the energetic high voiced ordinary church members. Crowned believers did their roles and were privileged to access clandestine affairs of clients meant for prayers. Confidential matters were reserved for secret prayers. While the prophets whispered to our ears messages received from God, the drumbeaters behaved as if the demons were taking refuge in our ear drums.

A thirty minutes warfare bore some fruits. My colleagues were already floored, throwing jerky kicks and blows, squirting the ground with foam from their mouths, their enemies revealing secrets why they decided to haunt innocent children of God, commanders of the high table ordering them to vacate, some even complaining that they had nowhere to go, soldiers of God giving no chance but ordering them to go to the sea. One who introduced herself as the grandmother of the victim requested to be allowed to pick her utensils and cigarette but the prophet who was mercilessly shaking the victim's head ordered her to carry her sleeping rags too. The girl woke up after some minutes of unconsciousness on the ground and with a sigh of relief, she heaved off the ground. She was branded a victor.

The mad man overpowered his saviors and took to his heels. Minutes later, he stood outside the fence letting out a stream of invective. The bad eyed boy had no drama but simply testified that he felt well. My case was cumbersome. I never felt any spiritual powers sending me to the ground, but one of the resource persons refused, insisting that my spirits were stout. All hands scrambled for space to reach my head. My eardrums were almost bursting. The war became more physical than spiritual as one preacher constantly poked my ribs with his drumbeating stick. I decided to feign success by throwing myself to the ground and with my senses upright, opening my eyes wide and systematically tweaking the pupils as if some satanic forces were being shaken in me. They asked my demons to introduce themselves but I mimicked the preceded casualty without metamorphosizing into a possessed being. They released me singing victory songs but I made steps backwards to nurse injuries caused by the assault in my ribs. I copied the victorious girl during closing testimony time when she explained how she saw her late grandmother flying away with her bag of rags but a slip of tongue, I named my granny who was still alive by then and bam, I apologized and incriminated my late grandfather upon rebukes from the preachers.

Humbug spread throughout the village that I was healed. Back to school, I maintained my position and worked harder although in doubt of my status. Wandulo was encouraged and he punished me severely after the District mock's results when I emerged number two. Sticking to his gear, I beat my opponent with a wide range in the end year examination and was the star of the school in 1988.

# CHAPTER THREE

Looking with bemusement, I accompanied Wandulo along the steep to the local shopping centre on his way home walking side by side as he nagged about my disappearance. I had gone to visit my aunt but stayed longer than expected. My calling letter had been on his table for a week. I accepted my messes, but his complains were extending beyond limit. Word after word, I remained calm like I would do to my parents, never trying to argue or exchange words with him.Finally, he gave room to my heartfelt question.

"Which school is it Sir?"

"It is Maranda High School, come tomorrow and pick your letter"

\*\*\*

## TWO BLENDS OF POISON

The deadline for reporting to my new school was blowing like Noah's trumpet .I risked being locked out if I didn't act in good time. A week before the last date, I had not known where my fee would come from. I decided to trek to the District Officer's centre with my details which he recorded and promised to act.

A month to the end of the first term, the deadline was long gone. My presence in the village which was raising eye brows toped discussions among opinion leaders.Okello, an area councilor held me by the hands and took me to a school within the locality. He introduced me to the principal-*Odundo* who admitted me to board while assisting to do a follow up on government funds.

The dark clouds of uncertainty hanging over my chances of education and health status were like two blends of poison mixed on my plate. I woke up one morning when we were in the middle of our end term examination and found myself in the same condition I was in the first time I experienced the attacks, this time in the dormitory, a foreign venue with no relatives to express their sympathy.

Lifting up my head, my eyes met the Christian Union teacher ; Miguda and a few students who belonged to his group praying and binding demons. Miguda moved his head closer to mine and started pleading with me to speak up but I refused after realizing that the assailant had sent me back to the pit of death. I felt frustrated, cursed, undeserving and a member of the dead. I started counting fresh losses, the worst being stigma from my newly found friends in the institution. I felt I was a misfit of the community despite encouragements from brother Miguda who kept on telling me how much God loves me. I spent the remaining days before end term in close relationship with the Christian union members in my lucid moments, the only group that could promise me life in despair. Their services had a polite approach, no deadly drumbeats, no prophecies, no candles, no special dresses but words of encouragement and simple prayers.

Back home, I never told mom or any other person exactly what happened to me but simply refused to report back to school in second term but to wait for the day of my last breath. Those are days I could spend whole days in bed. I became arrogant and always felt disturbed by anybody talking to me. Any moment I went into meditation, my face would be flooded with tears. My dad protected me from any harassment, occasionally he could sit by my lonely bed, chat with me, and remind me of cleanliness when he realized I was grimy.

The effects of my condition became as visible to the public as a wall poster. My sound melted like wax. I walked like somebody affected by partial stroke, my emotions clearly delineating my level of frustrations.

Weeks piled like a heap of leaves in dry season. Months turned like paper leaves. My schooling dreams faded. My classmates, the very lot I proved wrong in book work were making huge steps ahead of me, talking wonders when they met during school holidays, forcing me to turn my face in a grimace of pain, cursing the devil, I wished he killed me, than letting me walk with such a burden on my back and allowing me to enjoy the breath of life.

A boy of my age who belonged to another church of the vigorous drumbeaters invited me for another overnight prayers scheduled to take place in their church compound near our home.

The agony of presenting myself as a prayer item was cumbersome and bureaucratic. I made a surprise visit when the Pentecostal songs and dances were at the climax and joined frenzied throng of spiritual fighters celebrating redemption.

A prophet filled with the Holy Ghost sweeping through the crowd in an endeavor to separate wheat from the chaff pounced on me like a beast on its prey probably judging from my wobbling knees that I didn't possess the freedom I was claiming. He pulled me by the collar of my shirt to a secluded place to relay the creator's message. He heaved his chest as he forced out words amidst groans and shouts of praises to big Biblical names like Ibrahim,Mary,Gabriel *blah,blah*.....I accepted in fear of God's wrath that I was surely not yet healed. He prescribed some candles for the next prayer session and surprisingly, some token for the exorcists, the last message whispered with wisdom looks of mutual concern.

My condition forced me to imbibe the traditions of anybody who promised to offer solutions. I started following the church programmes and mastering their principles, cramming which color appeased which angel. I soon familiarized myself with the rankings of the spiritual leaders signified by varieties of gowns, caps, their insignia and accorded each of them the respect they deserved.

Having developed a strong belief that my status was a result of witchcraft, I developed a negative attitude against servants of God who simply encouraged me to believe and never touched on possible sources of my woes. I looked down upon church services conducted by soft spoken clergy who could lead the flock in singing hymns, read some script and wish away the day. I felt they were dismal spiritual failures who had no powers over devil. I became a good catch for the real prophets who could meet God eye to eye and bring down the message.

I had to brace myself before attending any evil battling spree due to scary incidences during performance by the God sent messengers. In the house of a woman who had invited us for the prayers, a prophet briskly climbed the rafters to the top of her grass thatched roof and descended with a tightly tied shroud of rags whose inside contents were unknown. He collapsed immediately he landed on the floor and started groaning. His colleagues warned the flock never to move near him. They explained that the charms he had pulled from the roof were more powerful than his spiritual powers and would not recover until a joint prayer was done by higher ranking prophets.

With the deadly object still clasped to his fist, he unconsciously shook his head in agreement to every word that was shouted by his superior prophet who refused to move near him but rebuke with a pointing finger from a distance with the rest watching in amazement. He slowly uncoiled his fist, let loose the object and followed his spiritual counselor who held him by the hands to a room probably for some counseling.

The incident brought all business to a standstill with the devastated throng of staunch believers viewing the object in fear from a distance like a powerful grenade and wondering who would have the guts to destroy it. Whoever would do it had to gain some spiritual mileage because it was a proof of the strength of powers inside the prophet.

The lead prophet resumed and led the congregation into a cleansing prayer before giving a formula for sloughing off the killer object. He gave orders for believers to move towards the object but instead, they made steps backward cowardly grumbling about the agony of getting into contact with the dark world's weapons. He requested for some paraffin from the host who provided by pushing a tin towards him from a distance.

"What if I decide to leave it with you here?" he questioned the embarrassed tongue tied woman who watched in disbelief with her hand on the chin.

He sprayed some paraffin and lit the object forcing the attendance to flee for their safety as if some teargas had been lobbed because of a belief that even the smoke from the object was harmful to life.

The more I came across such scenarios, the more my belief in witchcraft developed. It's still challenging to this minute whether they were true spirits of God at work or creative sleight of hand to win more souls by convincing them that God in those denominations was more practical than just words of encouragement.

A prophet who was invited to pray for granny one day when she was sick unveiled a nut after running his palms on her chest for several minutes amidst shouts of binding and communicating to his creator in tongues while our eyes were closed .He claimed to have uprooted it from her heart and went further to explain that it was planted by a witch to kill the old woman as soon as it started growing, an abomination to scientific discoveries. I wondered which kind of heart granny had to accommodate a foreign object in gestation and when a plant had ever grown by getting its nutrients from a human heart. Probably water could be replaced by blood but OK, God's miracles perform beyond human understanding. I imagined a situation of a plant's roots spreading on the inside walls of my granny's heart and shook my head in bitterness.

I saluted the prophet and became more of a spiritual navvy by assisting the anointed ones in carrying their bags to church functions and other unskilled labor like carrying benches but I never accepted to wear special dresses. This journey occupied my diary in the whole of 1989 with hope of getting healed as a result of my effort.

# CHAPTER FOUR

I sat in the midst of other fellow grandchildren paying attention to our grannies routine post supper story telling sessions always aimed at offering lessons in a way or another. This time round although not directly focused but the direction she was taking was slowly soiling my eyelids with a layer of guilt just like she had done to my female cousins the previous night when she told us the story of a girl who sniffed at all men when approached with marriage proposals until she became too old for any young man looking for a fiancé .She rued when she desperately ended up with an old lousy widower who was looking for an alternative woman to replace his late wife.

A woman who dies unmarried is buried behind the fence of her father's homestead to allay bad spirits of singleness from haunting upcoming girls of that family according to culture. Deceased senior bachelors would be buried with thorns pricked on the soles of their feet to gag the spirits of bachelorhood.

Granny's stories had more fictions than reality. The most interesting in my memories was the story of a night runner who performed in her home turf one night in the olden days when our fathers were still young. He ran and jumped around their compound occasionally coming close to their window, bashing it with his naked bums and farting loudly. Her hubby known to be a light sleeper was snoring abnormally and couldn't respond to even her loudest call. The night man who heard her calling went close to the window and boasted in our Luo language *"Ruben a bena ni to nyalo ang'o* (What can a mere Ruben do to me) "The night runner went further by whispering to her from outside that his charms had sent my grandfather into a deep slumber to ensure he snored till the night man accomplished his mission in the compound.

Having no alternative to fend off the dark world's sportsman, granny conceded defeat and decided to peep through the window slit. The grotesque figure in the nude had swollen to double the size of an ordinary human being and was bushier in shape than human. He ran around the compound in the bright moonlight singing his brazen song for the night's activity "*Bar……..!bar bia miyi mkenyeee bar……………!* (Branch……!branch come I give you my bums branch……..!).He went to the cow pen, untied them and rid on their backs. Whenever he alighted from one cow, he would bend with his head facing the gate and naked buttocks facing the sky, a lightning like light would flash from his arsehole torching my granny's house hence scaring our fount of wisdom whose man was dead asleep. He relished his witchcraft and could laugh loudly any time he successfully did a frightening lunacy. He praised himself with his underworld moniker; *Obuoch Oruka* (The Giant Mushroom). He concluded his mission by re-tying the cows back to their respective polls and jumping across the fence. Our grandfather woke up as soon as he disappeared and could not explain the cause of his unusual sleep.

My grandparents' foe lacked one important companion to facilitate his nightly activities no wonder he resorted to using his prey's cattle. Every night runner was always accompanied by a pet to facilitate the weirdo act. While some had leopards, others could use crocodiles, snakes, hyenas and other wildlife habitats which they tamed and trained.

Witch pets were empowered with charms to perform like their owners. An ordinary person walking at night could find himself in the company of a leopard soothing and brushing its skin on the victim's legs. The devastated pedestrian could find himself in a catatonic state and succumb to the powers of the charms. The beast could do all ungodly acts as its owner did to the casualties like licking their skins, jumping joyfully over the hapless catch and urinating on them.

Their wild nature were allayed by their owner's charms and physically modified to be admissible in a human friendly lifestyle. The sharp claws were trimmed, fangs were removed and any natural body weapon blunted or removed totally to take care of their clients. Reports from the victims revealed that while the animal was performing, some human sound could be heard in the nearby rejoicing. Very old night runners who could no longer go out for the exercise never retired but turned to hand held pets like tortoises, cockroaches and other flies. Keen observers revealed that they could isolate themselves in darkness and toy on the floor with the fly blurting out funny praises to them and giggling cheekily. This act is the origin of the old adage that the old night runner uses cockroaches.

The stories of human beings having supernatural powers gave us an excuse to use wherever we experienced defeat from our opponents in public arena. At the age of twelve, I under estimated the strength of a tubby little girl one evening on our way to fetch water from the village stream. I mischievously shouted at their gate with the pen name she obtained from her peers because of the rounded shape of her eyes and head. I persistently continued despite her tolerant silence *The owl..owl…owl….come out we fetch water the owl….!, The owl….owl….owl…come out we fetch water the owl……!.*

Irked by the gravity of the insult, the lady stormed out of her mother's house in a fit of pique, lunged forward and pounced on me with the force that shoved both of us to the ground. We rolled several times to a cassava plantation before she afflicted my face with bites and prodigious girlish blows that unleashed a spurt of blood from my nose. My attempt to overturn her failed when she sat on my arms dovetailed across my chest that provided a vantage for her unalloyed victory.

The girl pinched my bleeding nose and gave several warnings as I nodded in her honor before releasing me and detaining my water jerricans which were later collected by an older friend of mine. When I visited the boy who accompanied me but decided not to join in the fray for some data collection on the ugly scenario of an African girl on the chest of a whole man regarded as the kingpin by tradition, we piteously concluded that the girl's family could be possessed by the powers of the night runner otherwise, it would not be possible. In sports, we also suspected people with the highest velocity to belong to families of night runners. I secretly wished I was one because by changing the weakness into strength, I would be a leading world athletic champion.

In primary school one Sunday afternoon when we went for tuition, Wandulo found a monitor lizard on his office seat and alerted the class to kill it. None other than our classmate; Benard who was born and brought up in Nairobi moved close to the animal due to fear that it was sent by a parent possessed by the magic powers probably to bewitch the teacher for caning his child.

The octogenarian grandma explained that spirits of epilepsy worship the moonlight. They attack their victims every month at the onset of the moonlight to salute their god. They allow treatments of side effects but their actions are persistent. Treatment can be done by anybody with a medical solution including white collar doctors and clinical officers who know nothing about the spirit world.

I learnt from the acrid story that my attacker's timetable was shaping up. Unlike the earlier days when I could experience an attack after three to four months, they became more frequent and true to my granny's words, I would be harried once a month mostly at night. Her story also changed my attitude unlike my earlier belief that paper doctors were not recognized by God and had no powers to heal the sick especially in a case like mine. I decided to wake up the following day and walk to our district hospital located almost twenty kilometers from home for a solution to the endless pain on my chest and other parts of my body especially joints.

Standing at the hospital gate holding the packet of medications provided by the clinical officer who attended to me on my right hand, I felt a prickle of fear at the sight of a primped, brown and aging lanky guy across the road. The familiar figure was my high school principal in his spiffy black suit and glinting spectacles.

There was no hide out in the open space to facilitate my attempt to streak across the vicinity of his sight. I traversed the road to reach him. He pointed his nose in the air with dissatisfaction before responding to my hand that I stretched out for a greeting.
"Where have you been?" he asked angrily
"I am experiencing financial difficulties and am unable to raise fees for my education" I trembled while answering his question
"Who sent you home" he asked
"Not you sir, even now, am ready to resume if you can allow me" I replied
"Come to school on Monday" he concluded
"Thank you sir" I responded with ease

I sympathized with myself as I shuffled my feet on the way back home. The lump on my throat resurfaced .The quality of brain I had for academic performance and the stakeholders willing to nurture my talent. An evil sent spirit had firmly established itself in me and was proudly spreading its roots and claiming to own powers from the creator to punish offenders. Its wrath could not be compromised by any living being but by magic whose details were far beyond my understanding. If at all the saying of the oldies were true, I didn't deserve to carry the burdens of my forefathers long after they had disappeared with the winds.

 I wondered why after doing such a wonderful job, God empowered another spirit who works like His rival to monopolize the spirit world. His work is to kill and to destroy. It would carry me at will in a whirl wind and subject my body to fighting dangerous dead surfaces by throwing countless kicks and blows.

As a result of the attitude we had towards epilepsy and its related curses, I still refused to accept my status even at the most advanced stage and if for any reason I was to explain my problem, I always fudged the reality by referring to it as fainting sickness rather than *"epilepsy"*, a pill too hard to swallow. Whenever I visited a doctor for treatment, I always revealed the body injuries but never quoted the root cause of those monthly injuries that resulted from attacks until one day a clinical officer who had handled me for sometime raised his concern, I simply told him that I was suffering from fainting sickness. Since he had an idea, he hit the nail on the head that opened my pond of tears.

"Call it epilepsy" he advised

***

## BACK TO SCHOOL

Chirping birds from the trees above roof tops, whistling commanders of ploughing bulls, shouting parents ordering their children out of their warm blankets for usual daily activities shrugged off the night runners and wild animals who celebrate sunset and dominate darkness.

With my jaws tight with determination, I jogged away the negatives in preparation for my second attempt to join the secondary school. I joined the group of bantering day scholars who emerged from the maze of footpaths with doglegs on the main road leading to the school. I joyfully responded to their jeers by saying yes to every fun they made. They asked questions like "where did you disappear to? Did you inherit somebody's wife?". They called me funny names like the prodigal son and the lost sheep.

Odundo received me affectionately and directed me to join form one, a class behind my former classmates. Seized by the fear of night attacks in the presence of non relatives, I decided to learn as a day scholar, an idea supported by the principal possibly because he had been secretly tipped about my condition.

The school life accustomed me to daily physical and mental routines like sports, manual work and class work. I tried to battle with books to restore my primary school academic record which was deflated by frustrations but any time I held a book to read, my heart buckled under several questions. "Actually, what am I reading for? Where will this effort take me? What hope do I have with this demon in me?.

I found myself lagging behind juniors in class work. Miguda, the Christian Union leader was more encouraging. He would organize for some private counseling sessions with me. He assisted me in prayers. He gave me an alternative that could only help in day time attacks when I was awake but not when in kip, the name of Jesus is powerful and stops the devil from accomplishing his missions.

The assailant caught me unawares one afternoon just before the language teacher arrived for his lesson. Like drunkard spun by the powers of his grog, I lost control and found myself in a world that was rolling like a ball down the slope. I went out of my senses and about half an hour later, woke up behind the classroom. How I moved from my seat in the class to the place is beyond my understanding. Some soil had infiltrated into my ear drums. My face and other parts of my body were filthy with soil. I was stifled by severe pains on my chest as if some hefty load had been imposed by force from above. Bruises and joint pains ensued from kicks and blows against the ground. Something was pinging in my ears like a ringing bell.

I can't tell whether there were other viewers who were scared shitless the moment I lifted my head while still in turmoil. My eyes met only one village mate by the name Wycklif who also happens to be a nephew of the late counselor Okello. He whispered to my ears asking if I wanted any assistance but I made a slow Luo drawl to inform him that I wanted to be taken home. He lugged me on to his bicycle and rode slowly to the destination.

Uncle Steve's eyes brimmed with tears when he saw my wrecked body. I was brusque in my response to his questions. Even though not his talent, uncle Steve surrogated granny by telling me a good story the following day when I visited him at his home established almost a mile away from his parents' home. Seated on a traditional three legged chair in the shadow of a mango tree to feed his domesticated decoy quails that he used for trapping more from the bushes, he told me of two tycoons sundered by academic achievements repeatedly involved in a word tussle over a piece of land.

The literate tycoon was not good at invective but he could challenge his illiterate opponent by tuning to English. To avoid embarrassment in front of his three wives and the viewers, the illiterate tycoon could watch in dismay and shun defeat by continuously asking the only question he could afford to pronounce *"What do you has…! that I don't has………?"*.Amused by the poor English of the uneducated millionaire, a dry laughter forced its way out of my contorted face. A fortnight after the traumatizing experiencing, uncle Steve convinced me to resume my schooling against my wish. I went back with my head bowed down in preparation to suffer the brunt of ostracism.

Nobody ever told me on the face but I remained in suspicion of all rumors and whispers suspecting they were geared towards me. I became crabby and could easily confront fellow students whenever I saw them in group holding a private discussion. I confronted a huddle of giggly form one boys gathered behind a pit latrine one afternoon only to discover later that they were celebrating victory after successfully railroading their bullies into drinking juice contaminated with urine. I never dominated the class I repeated in 1990 as expected due to my condition.
Students disdained colleagues who had other natural problems and resorted to cruel jokes as a way of correcting them like loud groaners were told to sell the posho mills stored on their chests which operated only at night when the owners were asleep. Bed wetters were told to stop irrigating their plant less farms. Sleep talkers were told to introduce their dreamland audience to the outside world.

# CHAPTER FIVE

Buoyed by the spirit of success, my elated classmates joyfully carried their stacks of books to their next class on the opening day of 1991.It was a year of vaulting from bullied to bullies. No more harassment from senior students, no more *"monocotyledons"* as the senior students referred to form ones, no more crooked names, no more beatings. Instead, it was their turns to subjugate and exploit the expected new comers after form one intake. They had to revenge by applying the same cruelty as it was done to them while in their first year.

I was engulf in despair and remained broody as the joy of the new development swept across the school not only to those joining the second form but to anybody making a step ahead. I had to grovel even to the new comers for their sympathy any time I'd experience an attack. To me, bullying a form one was like biting the hands that could assist me in despair. I went to school without playing the truant as I did earlier hence leading to my repetition of a class. I maintained a close relationship with the Christian union members led by Miguda, our born again Physics teacher.

I found myself embroiled in the agony of varying religious beliefs in my attempt to knock at every door that could give hope who were indeed divided loyalties. Whenever I was at home in civilians, I'd attend to the services of the Pentecostal drumbeaters for some prophecy about my condition and the way forward. While in school, I'd attend to the faith based services that applied no tangible solutions but encouraged believing and prayers.

All safety precautions observed, I participated in all the school activities.Occassionally, I'd visit my books but never completed any page I started reading, a click of "where will I end up?" would choke my effort.

\*\*\*

# DOG SOUP

The arrival of beleaguered form one students was a ceremony to the established folks especially form twos who for the first time were empowered to bully their new juniors. Joining secondary school was a big step forward for any student. It was the first time the village pupils could change from going to school bare footed to at least protecting their cracked feet soles with shoes as part of the school uniform. From scooping meals with their spade like fingers to using spoons. From standing in salutation of any teacher who entered a class to just relaxing and responding to their greetings.

 The new development ensured no more carrying of reeds for fencing the school. Secondary schools were fenced with barbed wires surrounded by some vegetation to be managed by the groundsman.There was no more carrying of cow dung for smearing the earthen floors of classes to prevent jiggers infestation, all classes were cemented in the new planet. Instead of chewing sugar cane bought from the village markets, students would sip juice provided by parents as a requirement for boarding students. Incidences of fighting over top layer of food in the kitchen were copious in school.

The allure of walking in secondary school uniform was too addictive to the extent that even when schools were closed, some form one students could be seen strolling in neat uniforms and true to their ambitions, they won the respect of the locals. Village girls were just proud of being in a relationship with a *"jaseko"* (a secondary school guy).

The older students treated them as if they were enjoying privileges they didn't deserve. During meals, some culprits could approach a form one and tell him that they wanted to teach him how to eat with a spoon and while demonstrating, they could consume the whole dish and leave the poor student going hungry.

Some bullies could force the hapless students to accompany them to girl fetching missions during weekends and standing from a safe distance, order them to defy all odds and enter the girl's homestead and *'ensure they went back with the girls'*. A student once suffered a dog bite in one incident. Another was beaten by a throwing stick *(halabote)* thrown by the girl's father who aimed at his legs but hit his waist. In yet another incident, a boy was seriously assaulted by the girl's brothers.

I developed a relationship with the lankiest boarding student of the new team who was suave and sophisticated. He loved and sympathized with me after learning of my condition. He sacrificed to visit his granny who was a traditional herbalist on a weekend to explain my problem. He returned with a feedback that seemed to have some remedies. His granny had a solution but needed me to accompany him the following weekend. We borrowed a bicycle on the material day and rode to their home which was about thirty kilometers away from the school.

The old woman took me to her sooty grass thatched hut which was a haven for victims of various spooky encounters. She allowed me to tell her my story. She released me to chat with my schoolmate in a separate house while she was preparing my concoction but cautioned not to reveal the secret to anybody around. The cooking smell of some unfamiliar mixtures wafting from the hut was an indication that my work was in progress.

A beckoning hand from the spaces between the reeds of the door sent me back to the traditional doctor. She ushered me to a three legged traditional seat that was not visible to any outsider. She served a piping hot bowl of soup prepared from some flesh whose details she never allowed me to authenticate. The first gulp rolled back to my mouth with a force that unleashed even the stock of food in the stomach park waiting for digestion.
"Swallow it or you will not be healed," she snarled

My second attempt delivered some positive results. I hassled to empty the irreducible bowlful of nauseating content with difficulty and piteously placed my head on my two knees pillowed by my two open palms to at least settle down the digestive system with the strange meal imposed on it. I lifted my head to find my doctor missing but my schoolmate seated next to me. He was sniggering while fighting back a word that was about to come out of his mouth.
"What is it?" I asked him
"Do you know what you've just consumed?"
"No"
"It is dog's soup"

Pulsated with anger and frustrations, I crinkled my face into a warrior, coiled my fist into a weapon and looked straight into his eyes but lowered my stance when he informed me that it was the pivot of my recovery. By virtue of nature, the imagination of having such a crud in my stomach produced a wave of revulsion in my digestive system forcing me to puke all over the floor. The boy clicked his tongue repeatedly but decided to respect nature.

Back home, I never told anybody what I went through but formulated a conversation with our village herbalist. I alluded the story from being my experience and replaced my names with somebody's. I told him that a colleague who was a victim of the same problem underwent such an experience in order to get his comments. He fobbed me by praising the action and advised me to try and use the same solution.

I gave the dog soup a clean bill of health and became my friend's poodle. He explained to me that his granny was also good at curing occult miseries like *Sihoho*~a condition believed to be caused by a permanent gaze of a witch who sits at an angle and focuses on his/her unsuspecting prey for a long time mostly when the victim is eating. The waves of the magic move from the eyes of the witch like electronic currents to the stomach of the victim in style. Once rooted, they react by causing severe stomach ache that can even cause death unless attended to by providing antidote from experienced herbalists or forcing the suspected witch to feed the victim with milk.

*Ndagla*~ powerful charms believed to appear in form of plants. They are planted by the witch in strategic places like the victim's home and their effects are realized immediately they start growing, the effects worsen as the plant continues to grow and result in even deaths of the members of the home.

*Kingo*~Witchcraft believed to act when the witch picks soil from the footprints of the victim, mix it with some magical charms and perform the magic. The effects of the magic are swelling feet or even making the victim to be crippled.

Other solutions that my friend promised were charms for trapping thieves and night runners. I brushed him off one day when I experienced a powerful attack at night almost a month after the treatment. When I contacted him, he exonerated himself from blame by saying that am the one who vomited the magical soup.1991 maintained constant monthly attacks mostly at night making my condition to worsen even further.

# CHAPTER SIX

We supported one another shoulder by shoulder in our long tramp through the trail in the thorny vegetation uphill across the stream dividing the valley of two diverse landscapes towards the District hospital. Like me, Bosco, my village mate and classmate was well acquainted with the adverse effects of expulsions and suspensions from school and joined me in that regard to elude the organized strike by feigning sickness and visiting a doctor for documentations to prove our absence during the strike whose aim was to force the administration to introduce long trousers as part of the school uniform.

I maintained a jovial façade behind my solitude to keep our journey lively. Our way back was a glide down the slope contrary to the tedious uphill task when going. I felt gratified at heart with Bosco's decision. I survived in the school at the mercy of the administration and had no powers to join the others in revolting against the authorities for what I had never paid for, after all, only two days earlier, the principal had brought a cheque in my name from government sponsors.

The rough hazy wind blowing against us on our way back as we approached the school carried loud shouts of rebel students demanding their so called rights. We hovered in a bushy hide out at a distance to watch our colleagues doing their wacky messes against the administration engulfed in sombre mood. Pelting stones that caused damages like breaking window glasses and hurling insults at respectable personalities like teachers.
The celebrity photographer cut across the school compound in the direction of protesting students. With the belt lifted to the *'third floor'* of his waist, his hair designed in the old fashioned punk style, his trouser ironed to pierce stray flies, his sleeves rolled up in the Obama campaign style, he made huge steps at a safer distance. Every time he pressed a button on his hand held gadget, a suspect was captured. Business turned into misery when a protestor spotted him. He fled in the opposite direction and jumped over the fence to the primary school compound concluding his mission as a business gone sour.

All roads came to an end, the students downed their tools to listen to the principal who announced his verdict to a sea of pooped humanity seated on grass in the school quad at the sunset hours of the fateful Friday evening. All participants were suspended until invited back with conditions for compensation of the damages and some strokes as a disciplinary action.

Another incident that almost involved me was the day our cook; Abuom served raw food to students. He arrogantly told the students to cook and eat him if they felt the food was not well prepared. Irked by his response, the rowdy group jointly held him trying to squash him into the hot boiler. Although as a day scholar I had no share in the meal, I enjoyed the way he was oinking and found myself participating but I escaped on seeing the kitchen prefect and some teachers who rushed to save the hapless cook.

The wind of a student night runner suffocating boarders at night before the strike spread a frosty atmosphere in the school compound with every student whining about bitter experiences with the acrobatics of the witch.Odundo organized with some believers and cornered him at the climax of his work. It was reported that while performing, he could tickle the victims, urinate on some and did all weirdo acts from one bed to the other. His charms robbed the students of all their strengths and they could remain quiet like corpses in a morgue whenever he was performing. One student who raised his voice and complained painfully; '*He is baaaack....!*' Was nicknamed 'He is back'. He was famous with the name until he left the school. The night runner was politely requested to leave the school and join another as a day scholar.

\*\*\*

## CUTS ON THE NECK

I took advantage of the dormant situation in the school to play hooky any time I felt weak or ill and use the opportunity to visit spiritual healers and traditional herbalists. An old blowsy knock-kneed woman shimmying towards my mom's house from the gate one sizzling Saturday afternoon with the support of a walking stick drew my attention. Swaying around her waist area was a swag of unknown contents. We sat beside her to give audience as soon as she settled on a chair in the house and started giving grim explanation of details showing her profundities in my health condition.

The herbalist would be given a go ahead to provide treatment if her words proved beyond reasonable doubt that she had a solution but by the look of things. Her way to the next step was clear as my gullible parents nodded in agreement to her advice. She requested for a token as a routine before going into business, too cheap and affordable, a packet of cigarettes. She closed the door to cover us from the prying eyes of observers and spread a mat on the floor where we sat with my younger brother who was also ailing.

Our legs straight on the floor, all eyes on the shilly-shallying herbalist, confidential matters observed, we listened to her shaky voice giving the procedural counseling, spittle freely flowing through the wide six teeth sluice created and toughened by cultural teeth removers down to her chin, her piece of cigarette under consumption clenched between her wet tight lips blackened by a layer of smoke deposits occasionally releasing a spoonful of saliva carelessly splashed to the floor. She gave us words of life, murmuring soft endearment terms which were sweet music to our ears.

The doctor sunk her hands into the swag and pulled out a handful of some dry leaves. She pulverized them by brushing between her two scaly palms and equally divided between two mugs. She mixed them with water and stirred hence producing a powerful concoction full to the brim. With our shoulders slumped and our faces filled with sorrow, we bent our heads and slurped the insipid infusion loudly amidst praises and encouragements from the healer to allay anxiety. Lovely terms like *"sons of Gombe"* bolted our efforts even more.

Done with the first step, the second step was a little scary but we couldn't wimp it out for the sake of our lives. She requested for some razors. My bleary-eyed younger sibling already aware that parts of our bodies would be sliced bleated restlessly. Head awry, he resisted her attempt to position him for a cut. The woman whose services were offered in kindness desisted from using force and turned to me. Her knees exchanging swings in the sequence of knitting machine as she gently went round to my back. I remained pliable as she made two parallel cuts at the back of my neck whose marks still exist today. She took the same leaves from her bag, pulverized them and rubbed on the fresh wounds. The other casualty gave in more easily after realizing there was no harm.

The health service condition did not allow our departure before the mixture dried up may be to be absorbed to our blood systems. She whiled away time as we remained seated by picking another cigarette stocked behind her right ear where it was carefully placed to balance delicately and putting it into use.

I felt rejuvenated and prayed for proper digestion of the concoction we consumed lest I experience the same failure as the dog soup consumption bout, further more the herbal mixture was not as nauseating as the idea of having dog soup in my stomach.

Back to school, I became more active and participated in social activities like other students but from my experience, too much stress is a stimulant of epileptic attacks. A girl from another school who was a class ahead of me lured me into a false relationship when we met in a sports event. I played my cards as per those days by writing a nice lovely letter adorned with flower drawings lavish with giraffe height promises; driving posh cars while requesting for donations to patch my school trouser, living in a palace while chewing sugarcane for lunch.

The reply to the letter which came in my absence was received by a close friend who playfully decided to open and share it with others for fun having known that the sender was a girlfriend. My soul mate marked the letter with a red pen like a teacher marking a composition, underlining grammatical errors and replacing them with the correct grammar. In conclusion, she gave me a paltry 23% and wrote a comment *"Please try and make it to 50% for our relationship to continue……"*

I received the letter almost a fortnight after the official release day. My wily friend covered his ill deed by buying a new envelope and rewriting the address, carefully copying the handwritings of the lady but I smelt a rat when I realized that an old stamp was awkwardly glued to a new envelope.
I thought I was hallucinating the moment I opened the letter. I never believed it was the lady I knew or some cheeky intimate friend did it to spoil our relationship. Just before I gathered my wits, another student whispered to my ears how my friend unveiled the letter in my absence and went blabbing about it.

Seriously affected by pang of shame and stress, I shunned the school compound for almost a week till my parents intervened forcing me to resume. I never made any attempt to contact my girlfriend and inquire whether she was the one or somebody else but if so, why she decided to demean her future children's father.

My presence in the school was a nightmare. I felt like somebody had stripped me in public. I became a subject of ridicule. Wherever I passed, students would chuckle behind me. Some naughty ones went as far as nicknaming me *"23%"* .I was convinced that I had a jinxed background. I maintained silence in solitude and once more thought of contacting brother Miguda, for some counseling but that direction was also blocked. Salvation did not support such relationships especially with a girl who knew more profanity than the scripture. A *"heathen"* in short. To add salt to the wound, some finks had reported the shameful experience to members of the union.

I cogitated about my knotty encounter until I developed severe headache and other stress related diseases. A powerful attack sent me to the ground one evening when I was bitterly biting my lips while imagining what I would do if I met the weird lady who exposed me to public shame.

# CHAPTER SEVEN

The taekwondo guy throws his kicks and hits at defenseless plants and structures along an idle path as he strolls in his free time, he heaves and shouts commands of their principles. A naïve observer may suspect he is developing mental complications but alas, he is driven by the powers of his talent that will escalate his ambitions to the skies.

I slacken my pace and eventually stops by the roadside on my way to the office ,I lift my head facing up and repeatedly point the air with my finger in style, finally droop it to swing freely. Other pedestrians shake their heads in amazement wondering whether am mentally upright but relax; an idea has abruptly clicked into my mind on how best the first paragraph of my next article will begin. +

Be a neighbor of a single boxer and listen keenly immediately after dinner when silence prevails. The beats of *buf, baf ,bip and bap* may make you  mistake him to be a night runner jogging in preparation for his spooky routine but sorry, he is making up leeway on his punching bags in preparation to face his next opponent.

Our classmates who were preparing for the final examination in 1993 were engulfed in that kind of spirit.Watitwa who emerged the best could be heard crooning elongated mathematics formulas like a song he loved most. I adored the hardworking team as each gave his/her best subject a special approach mostly during weekend when I *"escorted"* my fellow day scholars for private studies done in discussion groups under trees in the school compound. Historians could throw their books to the wind and tell you the whole history of for example Fort Jesus and Kenya to independence without referring to any book.

Boarders would carry troughs half full of cold water and soak their bare feet during study time to keep the sleep at bay. The proud studious students developed what they called 'academic angle'. A walking style whereby one shoulder was lifted high almost touching the ear and the other lowered to hang at the same level with the ribs. They claimed that the lower part was caused by the weight of books.

The most hardworking students called themselves book warms/worms. I don't know which of the two words they meant but either of them made sense. They could be book warms because they kept their books warm all the time or book worms because like the worms inhabit the body and feeds on the food and blood of their preys, the readers spent all their time in places stocked with books and consumed the knowledge like parasites.

My visit to any discussion group would raise eyebrows although some especially those who had some clue about the condition that created a wedge between me and book work sympathetically embraced and tried to nurture and teach me as you'd handle a person with disability.

The going became tougher than I expected when my colleagues who were well armed for the exams started talking their dreams. It was a class of big people, the class of wannabe presidents, cabinet ministers, ambassadors and national directors. I started devising ways of dropping out of school to avoid the exams but reactions from my dad forced me back.

***

## THE BIBLE PILLOW

Brother Miguda's advice on using the name Jesus to keep bad spirits at bay worked for me and take it from me that the name of Jesus is real and powerful but it depends on your faith and respect to God. In my case, I met the misfortune when I veered off the spiritual highway and started fighting the air in the name of my estranged girlfriend. But even before, I was safe at day time when I was awake and could defend myself by rebuking the devil but when I was asleep, I could be caught unaware.

I became creative and thought the Bible which is also referred to as the word of God could shield me from night attacks. I developed a habit of using it as a pillow on our bed but believe me ,my faith was affected by shackles of temptations that result from peer influence one night when we decided to go to a village disco on a weekend.

The waning moonlight and the clear sky provided a conducive atmosphere for our journey to the venue which was almost five kilometers away from home. Armed with a big round headed stick (*rungu*), we joyfully joined another group who had whistled behind our home to raise the alarm as per our way of mobilization for such occasions. Our gang of pipsqueaks grew bigger as we slogged our way through by whistling behind the fence of every homestead to call more people.

The revelry was thronged by residents from the surrounding and neighboring villages. We kept ourselves busy yelling with other louses as the older attendants paid the legit entrance fee to enjoy the dance under the security of brute administration security team who cordoned the compound fenced with poles and fresh leaves. Our entrance trick was ideal but risky. We had to wait until around midnight when music was at the pinnacle, create an opening in the fence and creep into the compound. A dangerous attempt that could send one to the grave in case you landed in the hands of the paid security louts.

I slithered into the fence and lurked beneath the leaves when a leading record that would drive everybody crazy was in the air. One of our team members had already made his way in. I envied him creating disturbances with his killjoy dancing styles as the dancing couples smacked him wherever he mischievously streaked between them. I saw a huge swarthy woman who was unaware of my presence in the hiding sashaying towards the spot. She turned round facing me and unleashed a downpour of pee that showered my body forcing me to either take a risk by jumping out and face the law or stick to my guns and tolerate the prickly effects of the liquid waste.

I waited till she went and disappeared, crawled on my knees to a way out of the congregation and took to my heels, slapping off the urine from my clothes as I lollopped towards home. I swerved and barged my way past bushes and shrubs to force a short cut on hearing the sound of laughing hyenas coming towards my direction.

I lacked grounds to blame all the God's messengers who linked me to the spirit world. Despite their religious differences, they shared one belief; respect God and avoid influence of the heathens. For anything, I was carrying the burden of my sins.

By virtue of talent, I found myself enjoying our literature set book. The book I read without tightening my jaws. As a literature slouch, I joined the others in declaring my ambitions but with a different tone. While others said when they grew up, they would be some big whatever somewhere, I said I wish I had my health, I'd be a writer. Moved by the same talents that affected others, I could also be seen at times laughing alone even when I was not reading. Someone could ask me whether I was becoming insane but I could respond by asking for example; what could you have done in that case if you were Emenike? (A character in the set book).

The school typist who knew about my primary school academic records called and scolded me when she was typing our district mock results. She warned that I'd never be what I wanted if I continued shirking class work. The principal took a low profile because he knew the bane of my good performance. The end year exam results were as disappointing as I expected but I never cared, I had ruled that I was destined to die.

# CHAPTER EIGHT

Free at last from the claws of school rules and regulations, I sat under a tree in the middle of my father's compound to ponder on my next move. I was not worried about the poor outcome. I was left for the dead, good results were meaningless. I had no dream for any college or course.

Free from the surrounding of colleagues who were breathing high over my dying body, I felt more contented in the surrounding of coequal village folks who had no flying ambitions but today's food, shelter and clothing, full stop. They recognize and respect anybody who once ever stepped into a secondary school classroom irrespective of the outcome. They believe your presence is a boon to school kids preparing for exams hence entrusting them to your lecture. Local businessmen challenged in their calculations would visit me for solutions.

Somebody hissed clapped and shouted from behind on my way to our village market. The man shrieked jovially on his bicycle with my name. It was Wandulo, my primary school headmaster. I flexed my muscles to react in case of an attempt to inquire on my results but fortunately, that wasn't his aim. Wandulo wanted me to join him in the school he had been transferred to and assist in teaching. I wondered why he was still considering me to be a treasure with my distorted brain and tried to resist but he persisted.

I shuddered at the travails of being attacked in the presence of my pupils but threw caution to the wind and joined my former teacher as an untrained teacher. The allure of respect accorded and making a buck propelled me to a hardworking staff member. I binged on reading story books in idle times to allay my health incubuses.

In my effort to make the best choice of the church that I'd be attending for the Sunday services, I was confused in the shambles of diverse religious doctrines but settled on the Christian outreach ministries led by Pastor James and located on the show ground at the Siaya District headquarters, a distance of more than ten kilometers away from our home but for spiritual healing to prevail, the distance was no threat. A spiritual brother who introduced himself as Masha,a news reporter working for a local newspaper recognized my effort and proposed that I stay with him in his residential house located within the town centre.

A beehive of church activities dominated Masha's residential area. His immediate neighbour, Lumumba was a staunch believer and a member of the same church. A family of humble believers was formed in that plot whereby people shared all resources from meals to even clothes in some cases. We could share ideas, have prayer sessions after dinner, offer solutions to personal problems and help one another in prayers.

 The community saved me from the waves of bad influence and assured freedom from spiritual infractions. I left my teaching job and decided to concentrate in full time prayers. The worst challenge was how to reveal to my brethren exactly which hump was on my back and how to trash it. I had to be as white as snow but how in this nature? God sympathize with my soul…..!.

A cold chill ran down my spine one Sunday afternoon in a prayer meeting when an epileptic brother was dangerously thrown down into convulsions. Empowered servants of God like Masha,Lumumba and Pastor James moved forward binding and rebuking while some wishy-washy believers dragged backwards wondering what would happen to the hapless man of God. I disappeared to a secluded place away from the house and started fighting back tears which were persistently rolling down my cheeks.Masha commented during an after supper discussion that the spirits of epilepsy are too powerful and persistent that unless the affected takes the bull by its horns and sink deeper into more prayers, brushing it out is not an easy task.

A surprise visit of brother Miguda, my former teacher took me a step further. He introduced an evangelistic team that worked freely with like-minded denominations to spread the word to distant places. I joined them and accompanied them in all their missions but was afraid of giving victory testimonies.

On the eve of my journey to attend a crusade organized by the team famously known by the acronym, OFET (Osimo Fireline Evangelistic Team), Masha beckoned me to his counseling room and asked me what I'd do if I was told that a dear friend or relative was dead but I told him that as a believer who knew that death was our ladder to heaven, I'd thank God.

"Are you serious?" he shrilled

"Yes"

The message he delivered sent a pricking sensation to all the bones and nervous systems of my body. The team leader, Alfayo, a full time minister who ditched his job for God's service and his entourage were involved in a tragic road accident on their way to the crusade. All of them died instantly and the crusade was cancelled. I felt like my residential house had been stormed. My memories remembered some bereaved dear ones like Amieno, a sprightly young lady who would preach with her fist acting as if she was fighting the devil physically. I went on my knees and wailed loudly in prayers going beyond Masha's control. I slouched back on Masha's sofa where I decided to spend the night.

With severe headache, I went into a slumber in which my enemy hefted me down to the floor into strong fists. I lifted my eyelids to find a group of binders and rebukers at work. Brother Miguda who was leading the team must have revealed more about me since he had an inkling of my condition from infancy. They administered some first aid and carried me to the bed to recover.

My journey to Dr. Aruwa's (Alfayo's father) home on a bicycle seemed to be succeeding a fortnight after losing our dear spiritual heroes. Standing at the shopping centre of Got Regea, the directions given by locals and banana stems planted to show the way led me to the destination. Alfayo's body lay innocently in a coffin placed in front of his mother's house as if he was sleeping.

In a funeral service led by the very Rev.Bishop Wasonga and attended by elite Kenyan politicians like Grace Ogot, Alfayo was laid to rest. The other preachers who also died in the accident were buried separately on different days. A scripture read to the members of the team by brother Miguda who spearheaded continuation of the spiritual warfare encouraged people by narrating how Joshua took over after Moses' death and led the Israelites to Canaan.Masha became more careful when delivering to me the second sad news of the death of my uncle Steve a month after the incident.

*** 

## ANTI HOSPITAL GOSPEL

For the first time, I met a woman who testified to me how people who had suffered from the same problem I had were healed but unlike Masha's team ,her preaching repelled any man made medical solution. According to her, medical facilities are institutions established for sinners who do not have faith in God. She introduced me to her senior preacher,Odero who also resigned from his job to full time ministry.

The power of Jesus doing wonders in my new found church of miracle believers changed my denomination. Believers from far places could throng Odero's rural homestead and stay for days to seek spiritual healing. Enticed by the victory testimonies of miracles and wonders, I decided to stay with the servant of God with hope of being delivered from the powers of darkness.Baren women were having babies, epileptics and mad people were getting healed and so on.

My effort in the faith was promising but I hit a snag one time when one of the junior preachers in Odero's camp accompanied me to the top of a mountain for a prayer and fasting planned to go for three days. I discovered on the second day that I had been left alone and wondered how I could bivouac without my preacher in the wilderness with the slew of wildlife. The surreal sight of snakes, monkeys and baboons were too graceless and scary. I thought of surrendering back to our host sister in Christ but the fear of God's wrath being the progenitor of the prayer mission held me tight. The situation was worsened by a frosty weather of continuous scattered sleet and snow showers.

I spent the rest of the day bitterly regretting my decision in a prayer of tears freely flowing down my cheeks and made it to the following morning when I went back to our host feeling proppy and sickly. My spiritual sister who appreciated my effort told me that the preacher went back the same day at sunset hours, relieved himself and wished her a good night. He never gave any good reason for reneging on our agreement.

A powerful force whisked me away from my seat and slung me to the table my host was busy arranging for my opening breakfast. I heard her screaming on her way out before my memories disappeared to the infinity. The incident was frowned upon by the bitchy miracle believers who heard about it. The runaway preacher reprimanded me in parables for going to fish and coming back with a frog.

The second incident happened in a crusade when I joined another preacher to assist him in his vestry. I woke up in the morning and found myself on a separate bed with body injuries proving that something was amiss. It was a shame to be a victim in a congregation of people whose testimonies were infused with victory. I became desolate and isolate. When a third incident happened in another crusade, it was the first time I ever contemplated suicide. I was pilloried by all the miracle believers for bodging up their faith. Some avoided me like somebody infected by a contagious disease.

Failure to go to hospital any time I was attacked caused more damages. I was not an island in this pool of miracle believers whose faith indeed did wonders. There were some who experienced challenges but never testified openly. Some could occasionally sneak to hospital according to whispers behind the pulpit and others even visited traditional herbalists.

A young preacher one Sunday collapsed from the pulpit while in action and when taken to hospital, he was confirmed dead. Reliable sources revealed that he had visited a herbalist the previous day when he developed health complications and the attack was God's verdict. An elderly pastor described him as a dog that vomits and leaks its vomit.

Some cheeky heathens shrouded in a shrub a short distance from our venue of a night crusade threw a toy snake to the pulpit from where a preacher was bashing out victory testimonies blended with biblical phrases purposely to challenge his statement that a servant of God will never be scared at the sight of a snake. The preacher's Bible flew to the air as he jumped over the table leaving his addled followers to run helter-skelter for their dear lives. He later reconciled his statements with the situation to allay disapproval from the evil sent non believers.

In another incident one sweltering afternoon as I shambled besides Odero on our way to encourage a new convert who was miraculously healed through his prayers, the head of a doozy black mamba jutted over a wodge of dry leaves in a fallow land adjoining the path we were using.
*"I ba ba ba ba……………ind!"* Odero croaked incoherently making a U-turn and bolted on his toes, his voice quivering with fear.

Our Bibles went sprawling on the ground while we scampered down towards the stream. We stood at a safer distance to analyze the reptile's intention only to realize that the bruising experience was beyond our faith. My feeble knees tottered as I stood wondering what next. Terrified birds gathered on the surrounding trees were trilling in question of the devil's intention.

With a substantial girth and a length of about three metres, glittering black skin and mouth distended to the gullet with toxic saliva, Lucifer's field representative truly proved to us that it had what it takes to shear off the powers of believers. It remained unperturbed brandishing its head at the same point as if asking us to try and see. The mouth slowly deflated as it slithered towards a dead ant hill where it coiled itself in a hole curved inside the hill but pointed out the head for incase we would be tempted.

We lacked the language of persuasion to be allowed to pick our Bibles and resorted to prowling, picking them and going our way. Our mission failed. We went back to our knees to repent. The scripture we read just before leaving for the day's mission focused on servants of God who could step on powerful serpents but remain unharmed. For the first time, my preacher relented and encouraged accepting our weaknesses as we aim to be like God.

# CHAPTER NINE

With the binky bag of my worth hanging from my shoulders, I girded up my loins to fend off shabby street boys, robbers and conmen. No more drowsy surroundings with sleepy paths dominated by harmonious village residents but a hubbub of fishy busy bodies strewn with hooting vehicles and loaded carts. I stood scared witless waiting for the guy assigned to pick me who had not turned up thirty minutes after I alit, bothersome hawkers incessantly trying to impose their products on me.

I feigned toughness but the village cock doesn't crow in the city. I turned back and noticed a greasy weirdo street boy mischievously aiming his hand at my bag.
 I hastily went forward in a flying leap and decided to navigate the sketch map provided to reach the estate. Asking anybody for the stage was risky but my trust in women drove me to some two, briskly speeding towards a waiting handcart operator with loaded sacks of potatoes draped over their backs.
"*Todhie thiganana modo hoyo wee* (Let's go leave alone that man you…!)" The leading woman shouted to her colleague in their Kikuyu language.
"*Komaroks mbao mbao Komaroks……...!Komaroks mbao mbao Komaroks…..!*(Komaroks twenty shillings Komaroks….!)*" The Swahili crackles and whistles of a tout leaping dangerously onto a moving public service vehicle drew my attention.
I craned my neck and shouted at him to stop. They dropped me at a stage where I found my blood brother eagerly waiting for my arrival.

\*\*\*

## JOB SEEKING

Unlike in the village where the idlest youth is taken to the chief for grilling when a chicken goes missing, idling in your sojourn in the city is like dozing in a military camp. Birds of the same feathers flock together, a guy by the name Joseph who was common in his host sister's vegetable stall became my best friend. We would meet in the morning and wander around the Nairobi town looking for menial job opportunities. Toiling in a construction site for a whole day with spades and the weight of construction materials were good days according to us but bad days meant joining fellow unfortunate job seekers to lounge at Uhuru park discussing blank future dreams.

The vicissitudes of unskilled labor were at times too discouraging to cope with. The regrets of time wasted in class started torturing me early enough despite unfortunate poor health that blunted my ambitions. My cronies were a team of job seekers led by an experienced contractor who could easily win tenders. The kind of bullying that I experienced when joining high school resurfaced in the new fraternity. New recruits were mistreated and jeered by the doyens who would hurl insults and delegate heavy duties to their juniors. They were more bitter with academicians and would mock them by asking why their class work was watered down to battling with spades and sand, a career that requires more brawn than the brain.

The worst tragedies ensued one Saturday when we were expecting our weekly pay. We jostled through bustling crowds to catch up with time and avoid our team leader's invective and possible exclusion from the day's work.Gody (not real name), a stout, grumpy man whose body structure was distorted by his reckless endeavor to take construction to fruition proudly trotted ahead of us. We rushed behind him but he sped up purposely to remain aloof. He halted on the floor of the incomplete wall and vigorously changed into some rags that he pulled from garbage in the store.
"Are you still waiting for your mothers?" he chastised

The site was jammed in the twinkle of an eye with usual laborers and job seekers pleading with Gody who had been entrusted with supervision responsibilities to consider them for the day. We tirelessly scooped and threw sand with everybody pushing and shoving for space till the day advanced when we were sure that our buck of the day was secured, all the jobseekers gone and the working grunts sighing with relief. The miscreants shade off their veneer of obedience and started venting hatred on innocent passersby mostly ladies by bawling and braying.

 A sicko who had been busy mixing sand and cement besides me took to his heels towards an alley in a concrete jungle ahead of our working site followed by three bobbies one of them, a lady. He got entangled on a barbed wire and fell prey of the government representatives. I felt a blush simmering my face on learning that the female police officer was also offended when he was blurting abusive words on pedestrians and never recognized her in civilian.

The premature departure by quitters to escape from the wrath of more victims led to more quirky scenarios. A stooping sinewy guy who was most verbal alongside the arrested was waylaid by a group of heavily built men in dark glasses. Our attempt to flee failed when they ordered us to watch them instilling discipline to the illiterate basket mouthed casual laborer according to their description. The sight of a strong man pleading for sympathy is more horrible and unbelievable than that of a corpse waking up in the morgue. They concluded their punitive action with a blow which sent him sprawling to the ground.

Gody who was deified for his good conduct at the site was not perfect as perceived. A group of women who were strangers to the rest of us confronted him as we traversed through Soweto slums on the way to Dandora.He deigned to slip his right hand into the pocket, pulled out some money that could be worth his pay for the week and shoved it into the hand of one of them.

*"Na hao wateja wengine?*( What about the other clients)".Another one asked in Swahili ,winking mischievously at Gody and pointing at us.

*"Sijiskii(*Am not interested)".I retorted on realizing there was something sinister.

*"Wachananako, na kanakaa mshamba..!*(Leave him alone, but he looks primitive..!)*"* She reacted and commented rudely in a low tone lifting her nose high in the opposite direction as if filtering air. We rebelliously dispersed to our respective estates leaving Gody and his trash.

To hell with the Gody and Company, I resorted to hawking socks. Although smooth and less tedious but had its challenges. A hunky guy of the office type emerged from a door on the third floor of a storey building and ordered for ten pairs worth One Thousand Kenya Shillings, well-nigh the value of my business. He requested me to allow him to bring the money from a drawer in his office and nipped back with the goods banging the door behind him. I pushed the door open after a long wait and realized that it was leading to alternative stairs to the ground floor in case the lift developed technical problems. The bloke was long gone and I had to beg for bus fare to take me back to the estate.

Another scenario was at Kikomba market after I had purchased utensils for hawking. A hulky grey haired man carrying a Bible beckoned me from the roadside. His angelic eyes lulled me into believing that a share of my blessings was in his custody. He asked me for a direction of a place he was to go but I naively informed him that I was new in Nairobi. He introduced himself to me as an itinerant evangelist and told me as if prophesying that an enemy had sent some witchcraft to kill my fortunes with infirmities.

The message kindled my trust in him and I responded with alacrity to his instructions. He requested me to down my bag in front of him for sanctification. After sprinkling some liquid contained in his holy bottle, he returned it to me and just before he could take me to the next step, an intruder shook his right hand and started testifying how the preacher had saved him from conditions inimical to development. The testimony gave me an incentive to release even all the money I had for blessings hoping they would be returned as he did to the bag. He resisted and inveigled me in to handing over all my belongings to the new guy. He sent me to a church building behind a jungle of stalls to bring a lump of soil leaving behind my properties plus money to the stranger. I incautiously obeyed his orders but on going back, the two guys had disappeared. For the second time, I begged for bus fare from sympathetic fish mongers to travel back to the estate.

# CHAPTER TEN

When budgeting, you do it according to the size of your shoes. I settled in a mud house in the slums opposite Saika estate a few meters away from the junction of Kangundo road. I soon became inured to the humble life in a community of low earners where we could exchange pleasantries and aid, but it wasn't a bed of roses.

On the heap of trash lying on the slope of Dandora dumpsite down to the bridge leading to Lucky summer and Gomongo were a group of sludgy crooks dressed to match their ground reclining on the grunge. Rays of the setting sun gilded the garbage surface producing a deceiving facade. The sight of killer robbers who emerged from the landfill and pounced on me was a bombshell. They searched my body and took all valuables, worst of all even undressing me. I regretted for having defied my neighbor's advice not to follow the site. One step away from the murderers propelled me to the other side of the bridge at a speed I don't understand to date. The verge of death conjured to me bionic legs for escape. A group of food vendors were shouting at me in the name of a common mad man in the area.

***

## THE KENYA ASSOCIATION FOR THE WELFARE OF EPILEPTICS (KAWE)

Stress from the painful experience invoked the spirits of my common enemy the following day when I was back in my house. It slung me to the floor and as usual I found myself well placed in bed covered with my blanket, deposits of froth on my lips and a trail of saliva drooling from my mouth. Some sympathizers must have done a good job but who were they?

A woman who happened to be my landlady freely entered my house without knocking and took a seat besides my bed, her gaze permanently on my face in a manner to suggest she was keen to listen to my voice. I greeted her but instead of answering, she requested me to give details of the whole story about my problem which I did with hope of getting the traditional doctors from Ukambani (her origin) who are accorded more respect back home because of the belief that they produce the most powerful charms in the country.

She advised me to rest for the day but accompany her the following day to wherever she would take me for some treatment. I never cared to ask where but followed her to a medical facility where I was surprised to find all the patients sharing the same problem I had. She introduced me to the clinical officer who took my details and administered to me a dose of some tablets that she gave me in a packet and a card with the label of the Kenya Association for the Welfare of Epileptics.

I reported back to the hospital as per the instructions for further medication and recording of the health progress which they did by indicating the frequency of attacks compared to how it was before treatment. The frequency decreased from an average of monthly to twice for the whole of 1996.In 1997 it happened once and for the last time in the whole year. My doctor prescribed to me *phenytoine* that I used for about six months. I've never experienced any seizures, glory to God, I was healed.

My decision to visit the hospital that had the solution to my problem was heresy according to the anti hospital crusaders. I believe that God does miracles but the brain that provides medical solutions was created by God. Rejecting man made solutions should mean doing it at all angles. The vehicle that carries the servant of God to his venue for the crusade is a man made solution. If he decides to fly by faith, he will lack the wings.

In the mid 1990s, when our preaching was at the peak, a pastor-cum-high school bursar invited me to his house to help pray for his ailing child. His approach was wiser since he allowed a clinical officer who diagnose the patient and revealed that it was dehydration. He ordered me to lay hands on the patient and prove to the officer that God is more powerful than his book work but I refused. He reacted by laying his hand and shouting at the top of his voice for God's healing but the child succumbed to the illness.

The pastor turned back to me and informed me that he believed his child was not dead but asleep. He went on by calling his child names and commanding him to rise up but alas, he passed me the following morning at a shopping centre riding at a high speed with a luggage in a carton followed by somebody carrying his wife on another bicycle. I confirmed that they were transporting the body home to be buried. The servant of God died two months later when he had just come from a thirty days prayer and fasting from malnutrition after eating some solid food.

In another incident in Thika, there was drama between a woman and her husband after he called a doctor to attend to her when she was ill. She could neither raise her head nor talk before treatments but afterwards she fought back asking why the husband allowed a *"heathen"* to work on her instead of calling her preachers.

The going in such denominations are marred by elements of hypocrisy and regrets where one discovers when it's too late to change your stand or lower your stance. A preacher in Siaya tore his school documents in the guise of declaring God's call more than a decade ago. The same guy came to me to inquire how he could recover the same documents from the Kenya National Examination Council a year later.

A spiritual guardian in a believers' church reacted to her brother in law who had been converted to the church. The new born spiritual baby was giving testimony on the evils he had done but when he began to testify about his relationship with the widowed sister in law. The church leader went berserk and warned him from the background to tread on his line and stop calling her name. Nobody knew exactly why but it was suspected that he was about to reveal some sensitive issues that would implicate the spiritual mother of people.

A preacher, who sometime back, refused to talk to me even when I had common colds, claimed it was a sign of spiritual failures. Nowadays he is one of my best friends. In the long run, he got married and lost his first two children. The very person who rebuked loudly when told that a church member lost a relative asking why death would occur in a home where there is a servant of God. He remained tongue-tied. He disappeared and refused to attend to his own child's funeral. He unsuccessfully tried to divorce his wife, then later backslid. Nowadays if you want to clash with him, tell him about the Bible

The intricacies of diseases in the human body are worse than harm caused by abusive words of mouth. The effects sporadically spread to the systems and organs inhibiting functionality and causing inglorious defeat unlike external verbal offenders whose ills have no effect to our biological systems.

The underscore upshot niggles me to date. The latest dream in record left me in tears. A group of juvenile classmates led the way. Each biting his teeth on the pen, triumphing on the last papers. I slothfully leaned on the locker in disgrace, expiating my messes by shedding tears. Before I wrote a single word, my colleagues were through. Some force incarnating God's messenger carried them through the roof to the skies, leaving me for the trash. Their kick off steps lobbed a chokesome cloud of dust towards my face, forcing my spirits to skid back to wake.

I lack the magic wand to shake, to clinch victory on a horse back. But disastrous circumstances destroy powerful ambitions. My blood congeals into a solid mass, at the sight of the so called "who made it". We shared the same roof sucking the breast of knowledge. Over the years, a line clearly delineates the difference between the sheep and the goats. "In poverty, wear the sheath of a tycoon…! In times of infirmity, have the spirit of a victor…! Granny said; if you feel your teeth are stainless white, laugh at the disabled, but if they are rotten like mine, please don't. Nobody is beyond disability. Amen…!."

**\*\*\*\*\*\*\*QUIETUS\*\*\*\*\*\*\*\***